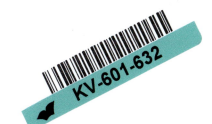
Guidelines for a
Speech and Language
Friendly School

by

a partnership of educational professionals from Swindon
including teachers and speech and language therapists

A QEd Publication

British Library Cataloguing
A catalogue record for this book is available from the British Library.

Published by QEd, Trent Park, Eastern Avenue, Lichfield, Staffs. WS13 6RR
Website: www.qed.uk.com

Printed in the United Kingdom by Stowes (Stoke-on-Trent).

Contents

Introduction

These guidelines are the result of a Standards Fund Project involving the collaboration between Swindon's Speech and Language Therapy Department, Even Swindon Infant School Speech and Language Centre, the Educational Psychology Service, the Education Support Service, and Penhill Speech and Language Centre.

Working together, the guidelines were developed to help schools provide inclusive education for children with speech and language difficulties.

Specifically, the aim of these guidelines is to:
- develop a model for good practice in teaching children with speech and language difficulties;
- provide appropriate training for individual staff and whole groups in mainstream schools;
- provide outreach support and advice to staff working with children with speech and language difficulties in mainstream schools;
- enable the development of parent support and training groups.

The guidelines include advice, guidance on training requirements, and other resources to help in generally raising awareness of speech and language issues in mainstream schools, and help staff increase their confidence and skill in working with children with these difficulties.

How to use these guidelines

Each section of these guidelines should help you to improve your understanding of, and increase your sensitivity to, the needs of children with speech and language difficulties.

The starting point for the guidelines is the Speech and Language Friendly Schools Criteria Grid. This is, in effect, an audit of 'where your school is at now'. Completing the grid will highlight areas that need to be developed in your school. This is an ongoing document and it would be helpful to date each part as it is achieved. Once these areas are highlighted, refer to the other sections of these guidelines as they should help you to achieve a desirable outcome.

The Head/SENCO needs to complete the third (whole-school approach) section C and class teachers should complete the first and second sections A and B (awareness, knowledge and strategies).

The Speech and Language Friendly Schools Criteria Grid

CRITERIA	WHERE WE ARE NOW (class teacher to complete)	HOW TO ACHIEVE	MEASUREMENT/OUTCOME	RESPONSIBILITY (school to complete)
AWARENESS and KNOWLEDGE 1. Basic understanding of typical speech and language development.		• Information filed with SENCO. • Training. • Encourage in-house staff development. • Information in 'Development' section. • Refer to Entitlement Document.	Teacher knows where to find information and has received training.	
2. Understanding speech and language difficulties. a) Understanding of terminology related to speech and language difficulties.		• Information in Glossary. • Training.	Teacher understands basic terminology used in relation to speech and language.	
b) Teacher aware of indicators of speech and language difficulties.		• Training. • Encourage staff development. • Collaborative work with speech and language therapist (SLT) and teachers. • Information in 'Development' and 'Checklist' sections. • Refer to Entitlement Document.	Teacher more confident in recognising child with speech and language difficulties.	
c) Staff aware of how speech and language difficulties impact on literacy development.		• Training. • Working with SLT and outreach team. • Whole-school approach/understanding - information shared.	Teacher understands interrelationship between speech, language and literacy and appropriate forms of support and it's use.	
d) Staff aware of how speech and language difficulties affect access to curriculum.		• Training. • Working with SLT and outreach team. • Whole-school approach/understanding - information shared. • Guidelines in school SEN policy.	Teacher has growing awareness of child's difficulties in relation to school curriculum.	
e) Staff aware of how speech and language difficulties affect social and emotional development.		• Training. • Working with SLT and outreach team.	Staff more aware of speech and language difficulties and their effects.	

The Speech and Language Friendly Schools Criteria Grid

CRITERIA	WHERE WE ARE NOW (class teacher to complete)	HOW TO ACHIEVE	MEASUREMENT/OUTCOME	RESPONSIBILITY (school to complete)
STRATEGIES				
1. Staff can identify how curriculum can be modified for child with speech and language impairment (differentiation).		• Training. • Working with SLT and outreach team. • Information in 'Strategies'.	Curriculum more accessible to children with speech and language difficulties.	
2. Staff can set suitable targets and write appropriate IEPs – share these with parents.		• Information in 'IEP' section.	IEPs have SMART speech and language targets.	
3. Staff are aware of range of specific strategies which can help children with speech and language difficulties to access the curriculum – e.g. visual strategies etc.		• Training (e.g. adult language signing, visual clues etc.). • Information in 'Strategies' section.	Curriculum more accessible to children with speech and language difficulties.	
4. Staff are aware of general strategies to promote communication – e.g. a) classroom environment b) teaching styles c) use of classroom support and resources.		• Training. • Working with SLT and outreach team. • Information in 'Strategies' section. • Best use of resources/support.	Classroom more accessible to children with speech and language difficulties.	
5. Two-way communication is in place between home and school.		• Targets/strategies/achievements are shared. • Home/school book or similar is in place. • Information in 'Strategies' section.	Greater communication between home and school. Home and school are working together to help the child.	

The Speech and Language Friendly Schools Criteria Grid

CRITERIA	WHERE WE ARE NOW (Head/SENCO to complete)	HOW TO ACHIEVE	MEASUREMENT/OUTCOME	RESPONSIBILITY (school to complete)
WHOLE-SCHOOL APPROACH 1. Speech and language features in English Policy and SEN Policy. Also, if appropriate, it features in SDP.		• Review and adjust policies as appropriate in light of speech and language issues.	Whole-school awareness of and commitment to speech and language issues.	
2. Training is available to all staff including a system in place for cascading information from courses to all colleagues.		• SENCO keeps records of all training opportunities (notes on courses etc. as appropriate) and log of courses attended.	Staff are more confident in dealing with speech and language issues.	
3. SENCO aware of the referral route for a child with speech and language difficulties and this information is passed on to all staff.		• SENCO has an overview of any child in school with speech and language difficulties and refers child if necessary.	Children are referred to SLT as appropriate.	
4. Time is allocated as necessary for relevant school staff to liaise with outside agencies.		• Joint target setting for IEPs is useful.	School and SLT liaise fully to help child with speech and language difficulties.	
5. Whole-school familiarisation with Entitlement document, especially sections which relate to child with speech and language difficulties.		• Time allocated for all staff to become familiar with relevant sections of document.	Increased awareness of entitlement by all staff.	
6. Resources are in place to ensure the requirements of the Entitlement document are fulfilled.		• Money/staffing allocated to ensure child's needs are met.	Child is given the resources needed to help them access the curriculum more fully.	
7. Strategies used with specific children are shared with all school staff.		• Time allocated in school staff meetings etc. to keep all staff fully informed of child's specific needs.	All staff able to understand and deal with child's particular speech and language needs, especially at playtimes etc. when some difficulties may occur.	
8. All school staff/parents/governors work together to ensure child with speech and language difficulties is as fully supported as possible and their needs are more fully met.		• Full sharing of information and strategies to help these children. • System in place for sharing information between home and school – i.e. targets and achievements are shared.	There is a whole-school/community approach which ensures that the child's needs are met.	

A 'warning' speech and language checklist

Child's name _____

Today's date _____

Think about the child. Can you tick one or more of the statements below?

☐   Responds inconsistently to spoken questions or instructions.

☐   Regularly needs instructions simplified and/or repeated.

☐   Cannot draw conclusions from information given.

☐   Has problems remembering auditory information.

☐   Has difficulty sequencing events and ideas.

☐   Is unable to maintain a meaningful conversation.

☐   Has difficulty finding the correct word for something.

☐   Rarely uses sentences of more than a few words.

☐   Uses sentences that are grammatically immature.

☐   Cannot discuss what is likely to happen in familiar events.

☐   Is particularly reluctant to ask and/or answer questions with an adult.

☐   Has problems recounting events, retelling stories, etc.

☐   Produces a short sentence at a time without linking information together with words such as 'and', 'because' or 'but'.

☐   Says little to anyone; does not initiate contact with other children.

☐   Has unusual/odd interactions with adults and/or other children.

☐   During playtime stays on sidelines or with an adult.

☐   Cannot describe how he/she is feeling or attribute feelings to others.

☐   Shows extensive hesitancy and/or repetition of sounds, syllables and words when talking (stammering).

☐   Uses the wrong speech sounds when talking.

What now?

- Can the ticks be linked to a particular area of difficulty? (see the 'Typical speech and language development' section).
- Can you find a reason for the difficulties?
- How significant are the difficulties compared to other children's abilities?
- Are other factors involved, e.g. hearing, behaviour?
- Can you find strategies to try in the 'Classroom strategies' section?
- Do you need to refer to speech and language therapy for assessment and advice? If 'yes' go to Referral form in the Appendix (page 47).

(with acknowledgement to SENJIT)

Typical speech and language development

Some children, although following a recognised developmental pattern, take a longer period of time to develop speech and language skills than expected. These children are described as having a **speech and/or language delay**.

Other children take a longer period of time to develop speech and language skills than expected and do not follow a typical developmental pattern. These children are described as having a **specific speech and/or language impairment**.

Communication can be broken down into three key areas:
- **comprehension** (receptive language, understanding);
- **expression** (use of words and sentences);
- **speech** (pronunciation).

Areas that affect speech and language development include **play**, **attention and listening, auditory memory** and **organisation/sequencing**.

The following tables outline the main stages that children progress through in speech and language development.

1 is a basic level, and children typically progress through the subsequent levels that are more developmentally advanced and complex. The levels do not relate to specific ages; they are numbered to guide you through the sequence in which children develop skills in each area. Earlier levels need to be considered when teaching because a child will not grasp a more developmentally advanced idea if he/she has not yet got it established at a basic level. For example, a child is unlikely to understand 'Which is heavier?' if he/she has not yet understood other more basic 'size' concepts such as 'heavy', 'little', 'long'.

If the warning checklist highlights an area of difficulty, you may want to assess what developmental level the child is at in that area and then plan how you can help him/her develop from there. The 'Individual education plans' section contains sample targets for most of the areas described.

Associated skills

Play skills

Development of symbolism

1. Plays with real-sized items, e.g. brush.

2. Plays with model items, e.g. tea set.

3. Represents real items with unrelated items, e.g. a box is a boat.

4. Uses role play with pretend items, e.g. a box is a boat and he/she is sailing it.

Development of creativity

1. Child copies what an adult or other child is doing at the same time.

2. Child copies something seen in the past.

3. Child role-plays and adds own imagination to what the person may do.

4. Child makes up a character.

Development of social ability

1. Child explores objects in isolation.

2. Child plays in parallel to other children, but not with them.

3. Child copies another child's actions after observing them.

4. Child takes turns and plays cooperatively with other children.

Attention and listening skills

1. Can pay fleeting attention to an activity, but any new event will distract.

2. Will attend to own choice of activity, but will not tolerate intervention, particularly verbal.
   Attention is single-channelled.
   Must ignore other stimuli in order to concentrate on chosen activity.

3. Still single-channelled.
   Will attend to adults' choice of activity, but still difficult to control.
   Child must stop play to attend to the adult.
   Must listen and then shift attention back to activity with adult help.

4. Single-channelled, but more easily controlled.
   Adult saying what to do during the activity helps.
   Can shift attention between task and adult.

5. Attention span is still short but the child can listen to instructions without interrupting what he/she is doing to look at the speaker.

6. Integrated attention – all aspects of this skill are well controlled and sustained.

Auditory memory skills

1. Can immediately recall what he/she has just heard.

2. Can immediately recall what he/she has just heard, in the correct order.

3. Can retain information long enough for it to be processed and acted upon.

4. Can store information for future use.

5. Can organise how to remember things, e.g. visualisation, chunking sequences of information, mnemonics, rehearsing.

Organisational/Sequencing skills

1. Has spatial awareness of size and positions and can fit together parts of something to make a whole, e.g. jigsaws, Lego.

2. Can recognise recurring patterns, e.g. colours of beads on a string or bricks in a tower.

3. Can sequence patterns from left to right, e.g. toys increasing in size.

4. Can sequence a series of pictures from left to right, depicting an everyday event.

5. Can relate activities to times of day, i.e. morning, afternoon, evening, and can orientate to the time of day they are in.

6. Knows the days of the week, the months of the year, the seasons and their cycles and can orientate to the day etc. they are in.

7. Can sequence a series of pictures depicting a less familiar routine/story.

8. Able to predict what will happen next (simple cause–effect).

9. Able to say how we know something has happened.

10. Able to say why something happened.

11. Able to predict what might happen next (several possibilities).

Comprehension

Vocabulary

1. Child begins to understand vocabulary he/she hears through regular routines such as meal time, bath time and play. The words will have real meaning and be of real use to the child, e.g. 'more', 'again', 'give', 'ball'.

2. Child may over generalise words, e.g. all men are 'daddy', or may under-generalise words, e.g. only one particular dog is called 'dog'.

3. Links start to be made between words, e.g. 'dog', 'animal', 'barks'.

4. Classes of words are formed subconsciously and a balance of vocabulary develops to include:
   - Nouns – names of people, places and things, e.g. 'Mum', 'bike', 'dog'.
   - Verbs – 'doing' words, e.g. 'jump', 'think', 'write'.
   - Pronouns – take the place of nouns, e.g. 'I', 'he', 'hers', 'mine', 'they'.
   - Adjectives – describe nouns, e.g. 'blue', 'pretty', 'big'.
   - Adverbs – modify verbs in some way, e.g. 'here', 'last', 'quickly', 'nicely'.
   - Prepositions – describe positions, e.g. 'in', 'under', 'after', 'with'.

5. Child starts to relate vocabulary to toys, photos, pictures, songs and stories, as well as the real objects.

6. Can sort items into categories, e.g. animals, food, parts of the body, clothes, furniture, transport.

7. Can sort items according to their function or attribute, e.g. eat, cut, read, cold, have wings.

8. Can sort into categories and sub categories, e.g. fruit; farm animals; cars – Ford – Escort.

Concepts

1. Child experiences a concept in lots of different settings and starts to recognise the essential qualities that must be present to make up the concept.

2. Child develops a basic understanding of a range of concepts:
   - Quality, e.g. like/same.
   - Colour, e.g. blue.
   - Texture, e.g. hard.
   - Sound, e.g. noisy.
   - Shape, e.g. line.
   - Size, e.g. little.
   - Movement, e.g. fast.
   - Quantity, e.g. all.
   - Space, e.g. under.
   - Time, e.g. now.
   - Number, e.g. one.
   - Personal qualities, e.g. happy.

3. Child develops a more complex understanding of their range of concepts:
   - Quality, e.g. different.
   - Colour, e.g. dark.
   - Texture, e.g. smooth.
   - Sound, e.g. high.
   - Shape, e.g. rectangle.
   - Size, e.g. heavier.
   - Movement, e.g. smooth.
   - Quantity, e.g. less.
   - Space, e.g. above.
   - Time, e.g. after.
   - Number, e.g. third.
   - Personal qualities, e.g. excited.

Grammar

1. Child follows one key word in a sentence. Nouns then verbs, for example 'the dog runs'.

2. Child follows two key words in a sentence. Nouns, verbs, basic adjectives, for example 'the black dog runs'.

3. Child follows three to four key words in simple sentences. Nouns, verbs, basic adjectives, basic prepositions, pronouns, early question words such as 'what?', 'where?', for example 'The black dog runs under the table'.

4. Child understands negative structures, for example 'Who can't see the TV?' and plurals.

5. Child understands comparatives, for example 'bigger than'.

6. Child understands more complex sentences and questions such as sentences in the passive tense or sentences using relative clauses, for example 'the window was broken'.

Higher levels of understanding
(The items below are not necessarily listed developmentally, but contribute as a whole to understanding more abstract information.)

1. Child understands cause and effect, for example 'Why is the window broken?'

2. Child is aware of what is expected in social situations such as when it is appropriate to talk.

3. Can take in information and make a deduction, for example can identify object from a list of its attributes: 'it's yellow, a fruit, you squeeze it'.

4. Can identify the main information in a story, conversation or instruction.

5. Can understand beyond what is stated, for example:
   Child: 'Shall I read now?'
   Adult: 'I'm busy at the moment' . . . meaning 'no'.

6. Child uses the circumstances in which something was said to interpret meaning, for example:
   Adult: 'Get ready to put your coats on.'
   Child: 'Oh good! It's playtime.'

7. Child interprets non-verbal information correctly such as intonation, facial expression.

8. Can interpret non-literal language, for example sarcasm, metaphors, sayings such as 'pull your socks up'.

Expression

Word finding

1. Can retrieve and use words he/she knows rather than using non-specific words or similar words.

2. Can describe something that he/she cannot find the word for. For example says what category it belongs to, what you do with it, what it looks like or where you would find it.

3. Can provide information about the sounds in the word he cannot find, for example 'it starts with ...'; 'it's a long word'; 'it sounds like ...'

Grammar

1. Uses single words.

2. Uses two-word phrases.

3. Uses three-or-more-word phrases.

4. Child develops basic use of grammatical elements:
   - Negatives, e.g. no, not.
   - Pronouns, e.g. me.
   - Possession, e.g. mine.
   - Articles, e.g. a, the.
   - Plurals, e.g. endings in –s.
   - Tenses, e.g. jumping.
   - Auxiliaries, e.g. is, are.
   - Connectives, e.g. and.
   - Questions, e.g. where?

5. Child develops more complex use of grammatical elements:
   - Negatives, e.g. has not (hasn't).
   - Pronouns, e.g. herself.
   - Possession, e.g. Daddy's.
   - Articles, e.g. an.
   - Plurals, e.g. irregular plurals such as mice.
   - Tenses, e.g. irregular past such as threw.
   - Auxiliaries, e.g. could, does.
   - Connectives, e.g. if, or.
   - Questions, e.g. which?

Narrative/Story telling

1. Child can retell an event, providing:
    *   A setting – the main characters, where and when it took place.
    *   An event/problem – what caused the characters to act.
    *   Ways of solving the problem – may include the characters' feelings about the problem and their plans on how to solve it.
    *   The outcome and consequences – may include the characters' reactions to the event.

2. Child can make up an event, providing the above elements.

3. Child links together events to form a story by developing the characters and their roles, establishing a plot and a reason for a sequence of events, and an end result.

4. Child links together events to form a story by:
    Time – then, next, so.
    Cause and effect – this happened because …

Appropriate communication

(The items below are not necessarily listed developmentally, but contribute as a whole to appropriate communication.)

1. Can make appropriate eye contact.

2. Can give a relevant and appropriate response.

3. Can take turns appropriately.

4. Can understand and use appropriately non-verbal cues such as facial expression, body language, proximity to other person, intonation.

5. Can use an appropriate speech-style for the person they are talking to and the situation in which they are talking.

6. Can initiate conversation.

7. Can join in a conversation appropriately and know when to stop.

8. Can develop a conversation beyond one turn.

9. Is aware of what his/her listener needs to know in order to understand what he/she is saying.

10. Can clarify what he/she has said when someone does not understand.

11. Can supply further information when asked.

12. Can keep to the topic under discussion.

Speech

Development of speech sounds	Age by which 50% of children have developed sound/s	Age by which 90% of children have developed sound/s
p, m, h, n, w	18 months	3 years
b	18 months	4 years
k, g, d, t, ng	2 years	4 years
f, y, s	2½ years	4 years
r, l	3 years	6 years
sh, ch	3½ years	7 years
z, j, v, th consonant clusters, e.g. tr, pl, sp, sn	4 years	7 years

Classroom strategies

This section includes a list of suggested strategies for the classroom that may prove useful in helping children with a variety of speech and language difficulties. For ease of reference they have been broken down into the following sections:
- Play
- Attention/Listening and associated strategies
- Comprehension
- Appropriate communication
- Expressive language skills
- Support

Clearly many are interlinked, reflecting the close ties between them.

Play

Play is vital for all children. It is through play that many speech and language skills can be learned and encouraged. A good speech and language role model at these times helps the development of speech and language skills in others. Some play activities can be adult-initiated and some child-initiated.

Adult-led

Try using the adult interaction approach:
- Sit with the child at eye-level.
- Watch what the child is doing.
- Talk about what the child is doing – provide a running commentary.
- If the child is not talking, copy what they are doing with their toys.
- Wait for the child to involve you in their play:
  - don't ask questions; don't make suggestions;
  - smile a lot and show approval and interest with your facial expressions;
  - when the child shows they are ready for you to be involved then either copy their words or give them a word for what they are trying to say;
  - then wait again...
- Adults in the room can be asking children open-ended questions. They can also at times be observing the child – taking the child's lead. If an adult is near a child they can get them to talk about what they are doing as they carry out an activity.
- They can encourage turn-taking in play.
- 'Helpful Hints' cards are useful for an adult helper – to show ways to promote a child's language development.
- An adult can help develop a child's imagination in the role-play/small world/construction play areas.
- The adult can also develop imaginative play situations.

Involvement with children

- Create opportunities for children to talk together through play.
- Having a 'buddy' system in place works well – especially during play activities.
- Create situations in the classroom where the child has to interact with a very small group of other children, preferably with an adult involved so that the child feels secure.

Resources

- 'Role-play' and 'small world' are ideal times to carry out this type of interaction.
- Using puppets helps many children with speech and language difficulties by producing a different medium to talk and listen to.
- Starting with the child's own interests in play activities is a good strategy to adopt – and then gradually move towards play activities you wish them to carry out.
- Children with speech and language difficulties need a lot of play as it helps them develop their expressive and receptive language skills in a very practical way. Play also develops their social skills and their ability to interact with others.
- Consider play in the:
  - imaginative play area (e.g. hospital, vet, shop);
  - creative area in classroom (e.g. modelling a car for Mr Gumpy, a rocket to go to Mars);
  - book corner (e.g. acting out area, puppets, story sacks);
  - language/writing area (e.g. using different writing tools/office);
  - construction area (e.g. building a bridge for the troll);
  - table games/jigsaws;
  - listening corner (e.g. listening to environmental sound tapes);
  - maths area (e.g. sorting different-shaped biscuits onto plates);
  - investigative/exploratory area (e.g. magnet investigation – senses table);
  - sand, water or shredded paper tray;
  - computer corner;
  - music area or a sounds table;
  - cooking/kitchen;
  - small world area – farm, jungle etc;
  - outdoor space.
- Think about other play opportunities you can provide in the above situations.
- Think about how an adult can enrich a play activity by modelling a child's play, responding to children's talk, repeating what children say.

Attention/Listening and associated strategies

The skills of attention and listening are the foundation of all speech and language work – they are vital skills. Children with attention and listening difficulties may have a problem following instructions.

Attention and listening skills

Instructions

- Remember that often a child will hear only the last part/word of an instruction so practise child responding to gradually more complex instructions.
- It is vital to gain eye contact (see 'cuing' children on page 25) – say their name and when they look at you continue.
- When you give a set of instructions, get someone else to repeat them (providing the child with a second chance to listen).
- Whenever possible, demonstrate an activity as well as verbalise it.

They will have difficulties developing their ability to listen and respond to instructions so:

- Ensure the child gives you their full attention when receiving instructions.
- 'Chunk' information into manageable bits and check that the child has understood each 'chunk', i.e. use simple, short instructions wherever possible.
- It is very important to use visual support for auditory tasks.
- Use natural gestures/signs to support instructions.
- Encourage the child to have the confidence to say 'I don't understand'.
- Encourage the child to repeat what they have heard.
- Help the child to develop a recording system.
- Encourage the child to visualise what they have to do.
- Encourage the child to pay attention in auditory situations.

Environment

Have question words displayed as a visual prompt.

Learning how to listen

- Waiting turns to speak is a rule that must be established and the listener should nod/smile/react in some way to show they have understood, e.g. holding hand up to acknowledge child and signal when it is their turn to speak.
- Rules for good listening are important and a 'good listening' poster is useful for its visual clues/gestures – sit still; look at person speaking; be quiet; think about the words being spoken.
- Children need to be taught how to be good listeners. Good sitting, good looking, good thinking are all important aspects of learning how to be good listeners.
- Reinforce this by praising children who are demonstrating the above (stickers/certificates).
- Have a code/magic object for the person speaking to hold and establish the 'no interrupting' rule.

- Teach children the rules/skills of good listening and target listening occasionally just as you target other things in a lesson (praise/reward good listeners with stickers/certificates etc.).
- Children need to give their full attention to the speaker (consider the environment). Avoid distractions both near them and if possible in the classroom and outside it.
- Gently guide child to look at speaker if necessary.

Simply starting speaking is not necessarily going to attract a child's attention and this is where 'cuing' children in becomes important:
- Get them to look.
- Touch their arm to focus them in.
- Say their name.
- Combining all three of the above can be most effective!
- Make up rhymes and songs to gain children's attention.
- Tell them what is happening/what they are to do etc.

Specific activities to build attention and listening skills
- Link memory skills to listening skills sometimes as both skills are important. The shopping game is an example – the child is given either a visual or verbal list of things to buy in the shop. They then have to remember them and buy the correct items (note the order they remember them).
- Play games to encourage good listening. For example, sit in a circle and say a child's name and then roll a ball to them. The child then repeats the action to another child in the circle (name first, then roll ball).
- Build up a class bank of questions.
- Have 'talk' partners and encourage the children to ask each other questions.
- Practise using questions that will lead to responses.

Memory skills
Many children with speech and language difficulties experience difficulties with short-term memory. In the classroom these children will have difficulties:
- following instructions especially if they are long and complex (see strategies under attention/listening on page 24);
- retaining information;
- learning new vocabulary (see strategies for supporting vocabulary on page 32);
- learning rote sequences.

Sequencing
Children may have difficulties with:
- word order in sentences;
- retelling stories/events;
- describing series of actions;
- time language (before/after etc.);
- rote sequencing (days of week etc.);
- following sequence of instructions.

The following strategies can help:

Vocabulary of sequencing

- Teach children the words 'first', 'then', 'last' and consistently use them when explaining the order of something.
- Teach time vocabulary in a systematic way.
- Sequencing helps children to understand language. Use 'before', 'after', 'next', 'between', 'last' etc.

Sequencing activities

- Do sequences using pictures.
- Demonstrate/have pictures to show sequence of actions.
- Cut up sentences and reorder them so that they make sense.
- Use sequencing cards – stories and activities in pictures.

Sequencing for class activities

- Use a timeline in class for the week/month. Mark on events, both regular and special.
- Use visual schedules to reinforce left to right sequencing (or top to bottom), but left to right is vital for reading/writing.
- Sequencing cards are useful for activities the child may find difficulty with, e.g. changing for PE. A book of photographs or symbol book for stages of dressing is helpful.
- Use sequence cards when a child explains what they have done/will do. It will help them explain their activity in the correct sequence.
- Using cards takes the pressure off the child – they act as an aide-memoire for them.

Sequencing and music

- Music sequencing skills are a good reinforcement activity. For example, tap tambourine, then triangle, then blow whistle. The child then tries to follow the sequence.
- Use picture cards, symbols, sequences to make up a rhythm.

Comprehension

Acquiring receptive language skills is another vital part of a child's speech and language development. Receptive language is the ability to understand what is said including vocabulary, grammar, instructions, stories etc.

Using visual support

- Use symbols.
- Use signs and gestures.
- Use real objects where possible. For example, hold the object up for children to see (such as fruit) when talking about it.
- Use photographs, e.g. the sequence 'changing for PE' photographs.
- Use pictures from books or computer programs.
- Gain attention to ensure they look at you when you talk to them.
- Use video.
- Demonstrate activities.
- Use visual/kinaesthetic teaching wherever possible. For example, an apparatus like Numicon helps children gain an understanding of numeracy.

Adapting adult language

- Use repetition – use the same style/language/phrases when giving instructions.
- Try not to change the wording you use.
- Speak at a slower rate with pauses.
- Don't be afraid of silence.
- Simplify/shorten the message.
- Emphasise key words.
- Wait longer for children to initiate or respond.
- Don't ask too many questions.
- Slow down the pace of activities as well as language.
- Simplify language – use simple words.

Supporting structure and routine

- Having clearly defined, labelled areas for activities can be useful.
- Having a structure to the session will help.
- Naming times of the session helps children know where they are and helps with sequencing of events.
- Using a visual timetable to support the structure provides a context and routine.
- Using signs to support activities such as tidying up and outdoor play is helpful.
- Support free play activities carefully. There is a balance between encouraging children to develop their imaginations/enquiring minds and stepping back, seeing the value of *silence*, and letting children discover for themselves.

Appropriate communication

In order to communicate and interact with peers and adults, children require a set of skills. These include life skills, turn taking, listening to others, answering questions, appropriate facial expressions and so on.

Communication difficulties

- Gain eye contact – say the child's name and focus their attention on you.
- Say and gesture 'Stop and Listen'. Encourage the child to listen and keep refocusing the child's attention.
- Break down verbal instructions into small steps (children can often remember/process only one item of information at a time).
- Use visual cues and natural gestures to assist with developing memory/sequencing skills. Visual timetables/choice boards can also help such as PECS (early Picture Exchange Communication System), for example, where the child points and fetches a picture illustrating what they want to say.
- Be repetitive when teaching new concepts/vocabulary. Reinforce both learning and language in a variety of contexts.
- Expand utterances, for example, add to the child's 'fire engine' by saying 'a big/noisy/red fire engine' etc.
- Encourage turn taking in talking. The adult should model this in play situations.
- Check if the child has understood instructions/questions. Have a sign for the child to use when he/she does not understand the question. Think why the child might not have understood (new vocabulary, too many words, too many distractions etc.).
- Help the child to plan, do and review during activities:
  - before the activity, encourage the child to talk about what they will do, what equipment will be needed etc.;
  - during the activity, talk about what the child is doing and is going to do next, and what equipment they are using;
  - after the activity, encourage the child to talk about what they have done (use usual props/photographs to help the child recall what they have done).
- Help the child with their general organisation skills. Teach them routines and encourage tidying up in set places. This encourages the child to realise things belong in sets/categories (this is a crucial concept in the learning of new words).

Social communication difficulties

- Identify strengths and weaknesses – then be realistic and work in small steps.
- Try to predict problems, e.g. changes in routine, offensive mannerisms, obsessions etc.
- Build on existing strengths to compensate for possible fixations, for example, if he/she likes trains, use this in as many areas of the curriculum as possible to motivate the child.
- Teach child how to say 'no' to those who might lead them astray.

- Teach social awareness (when to leave people alone and differentiate between politeness and friendship).
- Teach self-help strategies (ways of managing frustration/ways to escape).
- Help child to learn by mistakes (use role play, model good behaviours etc.).
- Encourage belonging to a group.
- Use concrete literal language if possible.
- Teach problem-solving skills.
- Encourage tolerance.
- Provide structure.
- Modify environment (see 'Classroom environment' on page 33).
- Make rules explicit.
- Try to be aware of danger signals.
- Help child to keep to topic and not overload listener with information.
- Let child know if they do give you too much (or too little) information.

Interaction

- Interpret gesture, eye contact, facial expressions as a 'turn' in interaction.
- Interaction is a two-way process – all the class can help the child with speech and language difficulties. An adult may need to initiate some activities in a small group.
- Turn taking is an important aspect of this.
- A symbol, for example, a hat, may help a child to understand turn taking (when you have the hat it is your turn to speak).
- Circle time activities are excellent for encouraging social skills including interaction (there are numerous circle time books available).
- Situations need to be created in class where a child has to interact with a small group – adult involvement helps the child to feel secure.
- Start from where the child is competent and build on the skills that exist.
- Choose activities initially that a child is interested in or good at, then gradually progress to independence, but always within a structure.
- It is important for a child to have empathy with others, so a lot of work needs to be done on emotions and feelings – there are many games to help this (act out each emotion, putting it into context).
- The child needs not only to understand a feeling, but *why* someone feels that way.
- Listen, and encourage the child to listen too.
- Sometimes question gently to develop/encourage play.
- Practise eye contact in play situations.
- Use play/role play to help develop social skills and imagination as well as the ability to interact with others.
- The adult has to take great care not to dominate role play, or play in general.

Behaviour strategies for children with speech and language difficulties (especially at playtimes)

- Introduce structure/close adult supervision at playtimes.
- Introduce a 'buddy' system.
- Reduce the child's time outside so that part of the time they are doing special activities (with friend) inside.

- Develop one or two targets and ensure these are reinforced especially before going out to play.
- Talk about games' rules in small groups and practise them.
- Have simple and visual rules, for example, 'no hitting'.
- Have social skills groups/cooperative games, for example, three people with pieces of a puzzle and having to find each other to complete the puzzle together.
- Avoid 'why' questions. Children need to be asked *what* would have been a good thing to do.

Multi-sensory approaches
- Whenever possible, enable children to see, touch and smell to support vocabulary development.
- Use a VAK approach to learning, i.e. make your teaching **visual**, **aural** and **kinaesthetic**.
- Use music to great effect – as often as possible to calm and stimulate.
- However, ensure children are not overloaded with too many sensory experiences all at one go.

Using everyday activities to promote and support language
- Use simple, repetitive language during everyday activities like washing hands, putting coats on etc.
- Use the same language to introduce different activities each session.
- Create opportunities for children to talk together and communicate with others.

Literacy – linked to speech
- Reinforce left and right sequencing (use arrow cards).
- Use frameworks for written work.
- Set realistic targets for writing.
- Develop comprehension skills through reading using paired/supportive methods.
- Emphasise the use of picture clues.
- Develop phonological skills (use of *Jolly Phonics* or similar to help child to learn and recall sounds).
- Develop vocabulary.
- Develop language through the written text.
- Be aware of the child's difficulties with reading/spelling.

(See also additional strategies for speech and literacy in the Appendix.)

Expressive language skills

Expressive language skills and communication skills are linked in many ways to communication – so the strategies are similar for both. This section will give you some ideas about how to help children to express themselves through building up their vocabulary and also show other important ways to improve ability.

Expressive language difficulties

Model	Don't correct child's mistakes, but model the correct way of saying it. Expand on the child's utterance.
Choices	Through carefully worded questions provide the child with the vocabulary and/or sentence structure they need.
Indirect modelling	Use a statement that presents the child with language they need.
Verbal support	Prompt the child if they get stuck on a word.
Obstacle presentation	Set up a situation that encourages the child to speak (comment or request). For example, ask the child to set the table, but don't provide cups (or not enough of something) so they have to ask.
Create opportunities	For example, home corner, role play, telephone.
Time	Give the child thinking time to formulate ideas and express themselves. Remember, silence is a powerful tool and can be used to great effect. Use open questions, and *give the child time to respond*. Slow down your input to the child and allow time for peer group interaction.
Encourage active processing	Encourage thinking skills and consider how the child reached that point in their thinking.
Make the implicit explicit	Explain the thought process (listen; think about the information; answer). Give the child time to respond.
Commentary	Use a commentary to encourage joint attention.

Providing choices

- Enable children to make choices of activities to increase their independence skills.
- Give two choices (forced alternatives). This models the language they need to use to request something, for example 'would you like milk or juice?' or 'Is it a car or a bus?'

Modelling and expanding language

- Modelling – this involves saying what the child has said, but saying it correctly (model the correct sentence/pronunciation).
- Expanding – this involves simply adding one or two words. This gives children a chance to hear longer sentence structures and helps them to learn how words fit together. ·

Speech strategies

- Model, i.e. avoid correcting speech. Rather model correct production and stress sounds where errors are made.
- Encourage other means of expression such as showing, signing, drawing what they mean.
- Do not pretend to understand – suggest they slow down etc.
- Use home/school book to fill in knowledge of events at home.
- Take time to talk over shared experiences.
- Speak slowly and clearly at all times, especially when giving instructions.
- Always remember to value what the child says and show the child that you do.
- Check that you have understood correctly by asking the child a question and/or saying back to them what you thought they said.

Using non-directive approaches

- Reduce the number of questions.
- Comment on what children are doing. Avoid judging, questioning or instructing.
- Invite them to join in and take a lead. Make suggestions and then step back.
- Play alongside children. Encourage pretend and symbolic play. Join in and encourage interaction, both adult–child and child–child.

Vocabulary building

- Use topics where possible to build up vocabulary.
- Find pictures/objects to match words.
- Introduce key words before talking about topics in detail.
- Constant revision helps.
- Learn new words in categories using visual clues (real objects, photographs or pictures).
- Sort objects/pictures into groups.
- Do odd-one-out exercises.
- Make topic scrap books.
- Sort in various ways, e.g. by features (animals – number of legs).
- Clap multi-syllabic words.

Avoid using jargon as children with speech and language difficulties often take words literally and this can cause unnecessary confusion.

Support

The importance of working closely with parents and other adults that come into contact with the child should never be underestimated.

Working with parents
- Work together.
- Talk through what you do in school and why.
- Build in opportunities to talk.
- Look at ways to promote consistency at school and at home.
- Keep parents informed on progress.
- Celebrate achievements together.
- Have a home/school book/diary to aid communication.
- Share new topic vocabulary with the parents so that they can reinforce new words at home.

Working with all adults in school

Make sure that everyone who works or comes into contact with the child understands the child's difficulties and knows the best approaches to help that child, particularly at their vulnerable times, such as playtimes.

Pupil grouping

When grouping children, it is important to ask a few questions:
- Does the child work best in pairs, a small group or alone? Does this vary depending on the activity?
- Do peers with better language skills give the child with difficulties both space and encouragement to contribute?
- Does a 'weaker' peer let the child with language difficulties experience more success?

Support
- Always listen carefully to the child to show that you value what they say.
- Give clear models of correct speech.
- Use one-to-one situations such as reading together to input clear speech models and point out written sounds linked to them.
- Use *Jolly Phonics,* or similar, to help the child learn and recall sounds.
- Be aware of the child's difficulties with reading and/or spelling.
- Teach phonological awareness skills.

Classroom environment

Think about:
- the position of the child when you speak to the class;
- who is sitting beside the child? Will they be a distraction?
- the chair or floor space where child is sitting. Is it cluttered? Do they have enough of their own space?
- the table the child is sitting at – is it cluttered with many distractions?
- the child's ease of movement round classroom;

- the position of classroom equipment – is it kept in a consistent place and clearly labelled (using words/symbols/pictures)?
- possible distractions – the child may find it useful at times to do an activity in a work bay or similar (in a 'blinkered' environment).

Individual education plans

This section includes:
- two examples of formats for a pupil profile that might accompany a child's IEP;
- examples of IEP targets for specific areas of speech and language difficulty;
- an actual example of an IEP for a child with speech, language and literacy difficulties.

General information on IEPs can be found in *The Special Educational Needs Code of Practice* (DfES 581/2001): 4:27, 5:50–5.53, 6:58–6:61; The SEN Toolkit (DfES 558/2001): Section 5.

Pupil profile
A pupil profile may be used to accompany a child's IEP and alert all school staff (particularly supply teachers and new class teachers) to a child's areas of need at a glance. Examples of general classroom support strategies that might be included in the final part of this form can be found in elsewhere in these Guidelines.

PUPIL PROFILE
School action / School action plus / Statement

Name: ....   Year: ....   DOB: ....

Name of parent/carer: ....   Tel: ....

Address: ....

Background information

Medical/health (hearing history, asthma, etc.)

Involvement of external agencies (SLTs, EPs – dates)

Other information (attendance, family history)

Education background information

Pen picture (e.g. information from Statement)

National Curriculum levels (e.g. end of KS results)

Key areas of difficulty

Areas of strength/interest

Strategies for support (see 'Classroom strategies' for examples)

PUPIL PROFILE

Name: Yr:

Support programme:

Individual needs:
-
-
-

Classroom modifications/ strategies
-
-
-

Examples of IEP targets for *listening*

Targets and achievement criteria	Activities and resources
To demonstrate good listening by: • sitting, looking and thinking for five minutes during a targeted daily class discussion without fidgeting/swinging on chair on five separate occasions.	• Teach/make explicit 'good sitting', 'good looking', 'good thinking'. • Use 'good listening' posters as prompts to reinforce message. • Employ agreed non-verbal signs to reinforce good listening. • Praise good listening – 'I could see P was being a good listener, she was sitting well and looking at me.' • Use games – listening for deliberate errors in stories/ rhymes; Simon says; walk or run to the changing beat of a drum; follow whispered instructions; find a hidden ticking clock/toy, etc.

To demonstrate active listening skills by:
• asking speaker to repeat instruction/sentence;
• asking for clarification of a word.
 	
Observed on three separate occasions within a one-week period.
	• Set up small group situations in which speech is delivered too quickly or quietly, an unfamiliar term is used or a long instruction is given without pausing. Discuss why pupils were unable to understand what was said. Offer choices, e.g. 'Did I say that too fast?', 'Was there a word you did not understand?'
	• Model what pupils can say:
	  - 'Can you say they last bit again, please?'
	  - 'What does that mean?'
	  - 'Could you say that more slowly, please?'
	• Make an active listening poster with agreed symbols/ signs with examples of why language can be difficult to understand.
	• Praise evidence of active listening.
	• See *Functional Language in the Classroom (and at home)* (Johnson, M.) which provides guidelines on active listening.

NB See also 'Classroom strategies':
- Ensure speaker has child's attention (seat where eye contact can be easily made, cue, name if necessary).
- Chunk information.
- Use visual reinforcement (pictures, gesture, signs).

Examples of IEP targets for *auditory memory*

Targets and achievement criteria	Activities and resources
To develop use of strategies that will enable recall of a three-part instruction by: • recalling three items presented as objects/ pictorially/verbally on three separate occasions and describing which strategy was used; • repeating a three-part instruction to a friend on three separate occasions describing strategy.	• Practise use of verbal rehearsal (repeating items/ actions/instructions – to be remembered out loud/ internally). • Repeat instructions to a partner explaining sequence of tasks. • Practise visualisation techniques (encourage child to imagine him/herself carrying out the actions). • Play 'telephone messages': Child has to take a message during a role-play phone conversation. Encourage use of 'note taking' using pictures/symbols/ numbers. • Use mnemonics to remember a group/sequence of items (e.g.: **N**orth, **E**ast, **S**outh, **W**est – **N**ever **E**at **S**hredded **W**heat).

Examples of IEP targets for *sequencing*

Targets and achievement criteria	Activities and resources
To develop an understanding of the language of *sequencing* – 'first', 'and then', 'last' (or 'before', 'after') by: • responding correctly to story-based questions – employing these terms on three separate occasions; • responding correctly to instructions using these terms on three separate occasions.	Use language in the context of: • story-sequencing (during guided reading or using picture sequences) firstly using modelling terms: 'First C went shopping … and then …'; followed by the use of terms in questioning: 'What happened first?' Retell a story using picture prompts and labels for terms; • instruction-giving in the context of games (e.g. in PE: 'David, first hop, then jump'). • the timetable for the day. Curriculum subjects: • science experiments, cooking; • maths procedures; • sequencing of events in history.

Examples of IEP targets for *vocabulary*

Targets and achievement criteria	Activities and resources
To understand five new topic/ subject-related words (specify which) by: • matching word with picture; and/or • placing the word into the context of a sentence; and/or • explaining what the word means, demonstrated on three separate occasions.	• Begin to target new vocabulary before use in class. • Illustrate vocabulary where possible – accompany with a sign where appropriate. Create a visual word-book/ word-cards and pictures in the form of memory cards and keep in a credit card-style wallet or on a key ring. • Make associations where possible (function, description). • Carry out classification activities (sorting pictures according to different criteria). • Play games such as pelmanism with picture pairs or picture/word labels, word/picture lotto. • Carry out phonological activities (e.g. clapping out syllables, identifying initial sounds, prefixes/suffixes etc.).

Targets and achievement criteria	Activities and resources
To encourage use of more specific vocabulary in order to replace general/empty terms such as 'get', 'put', 'thing' by: • successful instruction-giving in the context of a barrier game with 80% accuracy (on the part of the listener) demonstrated on three separate occasions.	• Use forced alternatives: 'Is she jumping or skipping?' • Encourage descriptive skills using pictures and by encouraging use of alternative vocabulary when child uses 'put', 'thing' etc. Retell familiar stories. • Write out sentences describing pictures/stories with missing words for the child to complete (verbally). • Play barrier games (e.g. with identical copies of detailed action pictures in which one child places a counter on one part of the picture and describes this to another child who must identify the same part of the picture across a 'barrier').

NB Word-finding difficulties – all vocabulary activities will help the development of word-finding skills. A range of strategies will provide additional support to a pupil experiencing word-finding difficulties:
• give child time to think, reducing external pressures to identify word;
• offer help and, if accepted, offer choices for unknown word or questions;
• cue by repeating the sentence, providing the first sound of the word if this is known, providing a picture cue or sign, or providing additional semantic information.

Examples of IEP targets for *prediction, deduction, inference*

Targets and achievement criteria	Activities and resources
To demonstrate the ability to make simple predictions based on familiar scenarios by: • responding correctly to five 'What will happen if …' questions on three separate occasions; • predicting what picture might follow in a simple picture sequence on three separate occasions.	• Ask 'What will happen if you … - take an ice cube out of the freezer?' - go out in the rain without a coat/umbrella?' - leave a cake in the oven too long?' etc. • Discuss what will happen next during reading activities. • Use picture sequences and omit the next picture to predict what will follow (e.g. LDA *And then* story sequences). • Practise 'if … then' scenarios: - If you are hot, then … - If you find some money, then … - If your hands are dirty, then …

Targets and achievement criteria	Activities and resources
To demonstrate the ability to make simple deductions/inferences based on verbal/textual/pictorial information by: • responding correctly to five 'What am I?' questions on three separate occasions; • inferring information from text on three separate occasions.	• Describe a hidden object in a bag using appearance, function etc. • Play 'What am I?' - I am in the sky. I am white … what am I? - I have 4 legs, I climb trees and purr … what am I? • Miss out a word when retelling a story. Use cloze passages. • Ask general questions requiring deduction based on pictures/text: - The man ran to the platform and saw the train pulling out of the station. What has happened? - 'Help!' shouted Bill. Then there was a splash. What has happened? - The boy kicked the ball and there was the sound of glass smashing. What has happened? • Use LDA 'Why/because' picture cards.

Examples of IEP targets for *grammatical structures*

Before targeting a skill in a child's expressive language consider whether he/she understands the structure. If this is not the case ensure activities target comprehension of the target before seeking evidence of the structure in expressive language.

Targets and achievement criteria	Activities and resources

To demonstrate understanding of regular plurals (-s) by:
• choosing the correct picture (e.g. cat/cats) with 80% accuracy on three separate occasions.
	• Practise listening for 's' at the ends of words
	  - sorting pictures (sock/socks);
	  - listening to words and identifying which end in 's' (placing counter in box each time 's' is identified).
	• Discuss how the word changes when it is a plural – use words and colour to highlight 's'. Match labels to pictures.
	• Ask for pictures: 'Give me the picture of the cats.'
	• Play lotto: identify a picture by hearing word spoken only (e.g. pen/pens, fork/forks etc.).

Targets and achievement criteria	Activities and resources
To demonstrate the use of regular past tense verbs by: • responding to questions 'What did he/she do?' with 80% accuracy (e.g. four out of five correct) on three separate occasions. Followed by: • using regular past tense verbs spontaneously in the context of retelling a familiar sequence/story on three separate occasions.	• Play an action game (e.g. copy cat, Simon says, follow my leader etc.) and then name what the child did (jumped, skipped etc.). • Describe pictures and illustrated text using the prompt 'What did he/she do?' • Play games with action pictures in matching/lotto/pairs games. • Describe familiar sequences (e.g. 'What did you do this morning?' Washed, dressed, packed bag, walked to school etc.). • Reinforce verbal label with written label adding 'ed' in colour to reinforce tense change.

Examples of IEP targets for *speech*

Work on speech production should only take place under the guidance of a speech and language therapist. Targets addressing specific speech sounds will be aimed at reinforcing/generalising targets that have been achieved within a speech therapy programme.

Targets and achievement criteria	Activities and resources
To reinforce the production of 'k' in the context of words: • observe correct use of 'k' on three separate occasions when naming pictures beginning with 'k'.	• Practise production of words beginning (or ending) with 'k' using pictures/objects targeting the sound in this position in the context of games. • Reinforce usage in context of reading. • Provide choice when production is not correct: 'Is that a cat or a king?' • Encourage repetition of adult model. • Praise correct use of 'k' when this occurs. • Liaise with parents to reinforce target and praise.

NB See also 'Classroom strategies' about providing clear models of speech, not guessing or pretending to understand if you have not understood a child's speech, asking questions – using other cues if necessary (visual, non-verbal), using a home/school book to provide contextual information etc.

Targets and achievement criteria	Activities and resources
To speak with normal volume in response to adult non-verbal prompt on five separate occasions.	• Model appropriate speaking volume. • Distinguish between quiet, normal, loud speaking volumes. • Discuss situations in which you would use a quiet, a normal and a loud speaking voice. Use role play to practise skills. • Use a tape recorder or video to raise self-awareness and provide self-monitoring. Rate volume levels. • Use a non-verbal cue (e.g. finger over lips) when volume is too high.

NB: Check that the child's hearing is within the normal range.

Appendix

Speech and language terms explained

Alternative/Augmentative communication	Something used in place of or to support speech, e.g. computers, symbols, signing etc.
Articulation	Movement of tongue, jaws, soft palate and lips to make speech sounds.
Auditory discrimination	Listening to and identifying differences and similarities between sounds.
Auditory memory	Remembering what you have just heard, including the order in which you heard them.
Cause/effect	Understanding/expressing a relationship where one event causes another.
Chunking	Giving information in small amounts, one piece at a time, by pausing between each idea. Each piece of information can then be given processing time.
Comprehension/ Verbal comprehension/ Receptive language	Understanding what is said, including vocabulary, grammar, instructions, stories etc.
Dysarthria	Muscle weakness causing speech patterns to be abnormal because the speech muscles cannot be moved correctly for speech.
Dysfluency	Stammering, where speech may be hesitant, with sounds repeated, prolonged or blocked so that no sound is made.
Dyspraxia	Difficulties affecting the planning and co-ordination of muscle movements. This may affect speech muscles alone (verbal dyspráxia) and/or muscles of the body.
Expressive language	The use of words and sentences, vocabulary and grammar, and organising sentences into narrative explanations etc.
Key words	The main content words that carry meaning, as in a telegram, e.g. Put the brick in the cup.
Language	See Expressive language.
Language delay	A child may be talking in a way appropriate for a younger child.

Morphology	The grammatical words and parts of words, e.g. <u>the</u> dog<u>'s</u> bone<u>s</u>.
Organisational skills	Being able to know what you need, when and in which order. With language you need to be able to select vocabulary, organise thoughts into sentences with grammar, put the sentences into a logical order etc.
Phoneme	A single speech sound, e.g. eight = ay + t (two phonemes).
Phonetics	Writing how a word is pronounced.
Phonological awareness	Awareness of speech sounds in words and the ability to manipulate them. Includes rhyme, alliteration and spoonerisms (e.g. mad cat > cad mat).
Phonology	The speech sound system of a particular language – which sounds are used and permitted combinations (e.g. in English we do not start any words with the 'ng' sound).
Pragmatics	The way we select and use different words and phrases to convey meaning in different contexts and the way we understand this. It includes social uses of language, sarcasm, jokes, idioms, etc.
Prosody	The 'music' of speech, including use of pitch, volume, rate and stress.
Receptive language	See Comprehension.
Sequencing skills	The ability to place pictures, writing, events, activities or thoughts in a logical order.
Specific language impairment	Language skills may be significantly delayed in relation to other skills, or language use shows features that are not part of normal development.
Speech	The way words are pronounced.
Speech processing	The ability to perceive, discriminate and analyse speech sounds in spoken language (input) and to remember and select correct sounds for talking (output).
Symbolic play	Imagining a toy or an object is something else and using it in play, e.g. a box becomes a doll's bed.
Syntax	The way words combine in phrases and sentences grammatically, e.g. subject – verb – object (the cat caught the mouse).

Verbal comprehension	See Comprehension.
Visualisation	A strategy to help remember things, by picturing them in your head, e.g. picturing the things you need as the teacher gives an instruction.
Visual memory	Remembering what you have just seen, including the order items were in.
Voice	The vocal quality of speech which is affected by breath control and neck tension. A voice may be husky or absent at times during a throat infection, but should not be a longer term feature.

Additional strategies for speech and literacy

Children with a history of speech difficulties may find the acquisition of literacy skills problematic. They may have particular weaknesses with phonological (and phoneme) awareness: blending, segmenting, sequencing and manipulating syllables, rhyme and phonemes. These children will need to be taught these skills explicitly using multi-sensory methods.

Supporting sound/symbol correspondence

- Feel, trace and say **'tactile' letters** (velvet, sandpaper, wooden). Trace in sand, shaving foam, on large sheets or on the board. Make letters out of plasticine/playdoh/clay.
- Use **actions** linked to sounds (e.g. *Jolly Phonics*).
- Record sounds using a language master and the child's own **voice**.
- Practise with a set **visual prompt cards**. As a new sound is introduced make a new card showing the letter(s) on one side and a 'trigger' word for the sound (chosen or drawn by the child) on the other:

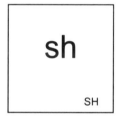 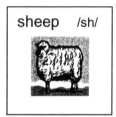

Supporting phoneme awareness and word-building skills

- Use **word puzzles**. For example, to build the word 'munch':
    - draw four lines on a small whiteboard to represent each sound;
    - lay out the word puzzle along the top in a muddled order;

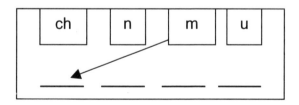

    - move your fingers across the lines as you say the word in a 'stretched out' way (not splitting up the sounds);
    - ask the child what they hear when your finger is at the first line;
    - the child then builds the word using the puzzle pieces – saying each sound as it is brought to the line;
    - once complete reinforce again the sounds and the word.

- Practise **phoneme manipulation**. Write 'stop' on the whiteboard. Change 'stop' into 'step' then 'step' into 'stem' (changing one sound at a time).

Additional strategies for language and literacy

Children with language difficulties may experience difficulties understanding what they read (even though they can sometimes 'decode' the text).

Supporting comprehension

- Identify the **vocabulary** that the child is not understanding. Teach using visual and concrete reinforcement. Place into sentences and check retention over time.
- Check understanding of **idiomatic/metaphorical** language.
- **Summarise** text and ask questions (pupil and adult).
- **Share** views about the plot and characters.
- Develop practice in **prediction** and **inference**.

Developing fluency and speed (which supports comprehension)

- Use **timed** reading activities (e.g. daily timed reading of a small group of words to increase speed of recall).
- See *Stride Ahead* by Keda Cowling (author of *Toe by Toe*) for pupils with reading ages 8.5+ but difficulties with reading fluency and comprehension.

Children with language difficulties may also experience difficulties expressing themselves in writing due to difficulties with vocabulary, spelling, sentence formulation, grammar and organisation of ideas.

Supporting writing

- Use **writing frameworks** (story plans and headings), sentence starters for completion, cloze passages (providing key words).
- Match sentence halves, order and sequence sentences.
- Encourage **shared** writing (with adult or another pupil).
- **Label** diagrams (providing words).

Offer alternative methods of recording through:
- drawings, diagrams or posters;
- flow charts and mind maps (e.g. *Inspiration* program from iANSYST 0800 018 0045);
- models or collages.

Referral form for Speech and Language Therapy Assessment (children)

This is an example of a referral form that may be used if you have a concern about a child having used the warning checklist. Simply fill in the details and hand it to the SLT department.

Please complete in BLOCK CAPITALS

Date:_____

Full name:_____

Date of birth: _____ Sex: _____

Name of carer: _____

Address:_____

_____

_____ Post code: _____

Tel:_____ Other contact number/s:_____

GP:_____

First language (if not English):_____

Interpreter required?   Yes / No

For pre-school child

Goes to pre-school at: _____

Sessions attended: _____

Name of contact:_____

Code of Practice: action / action plus / undergoing statutory assessment / Statement / none

Preferred school:_____

School start date: _____

For school child

School: _____

School year: _____

Class teacher: _____

SENCO:_____

Code of Practice: action / action plus / undergoing statutory assessment / Statement / none

---

Reason for referral

_____

_____

Medical/developmental information

_____

_____

Hearing test result and date

_____

_____

Other professionals involved

_____

_____

Other information

_____

_____

Details of referrer

Name: _____

Designation: _____

Address: _____

Tel: _____

Name of Health Visitor: _____ Base: _____

Please sign to confirm that you have obtained parent/carer permission for this referral, and ask for a signature if possible.

Parent/Carer's signature: _____ Date: _____

Referrer's signature: _____ Date: _____

_____

Information for Speech and Language Therapist from school/pre-school

1) Nature of difficulty with communication and effect on accessing the curriculum in terms of:

   (a) Child's understanding/comprehension of spoken language

   _____

   _____

   _____

   (b) Expressing him/herself in spoken words and sentences

   _____

   _____

   _____

   (c) Pronunciation (speech sound errors), clarity of speech

   _____

   _____

   _____

   (d) Stammering

   _____

   _____

   _____

   (e) Interaction with other people

   _____

   _____

   _____

2) Child's strengths

   _____

   _____

   _____

   _____

3) Please say what you need from this speech and langauge therapy assessment

_____

_____

_____

_____

4) What support arrangements are available? (Please give the name of the Support Assistant, if applicable)

_____

_____

_____

_____

Signed by

Parent: _____

Class teacher: _____

SENCO: _____

Examples of IEPs for children with speech, language and literacy difficulties

Individual Education Plan

Name:
Area/s of concern:
Class teacher:
Supported by:

Start date: September 2005
Proposed support: Unit provision

Stage: Statemented
Year group/IEP No. 6/19
Review date: Dec 05
Support began:

Targets to be achieved	Achievement criteria	Possible resources or techniques	Possible class strategies	Ideas for support/assistant	Outcome
1) To understand and use the irregular past tense.	1) Correct use in everyday speech on 8/10 separate occasions.	1) Reading books; picture books; posters; language cards; group discussions.	1) Talk about meanings of the words. Encourage correct use when discussing pictures etc.	1) Model correct use. Encourage correct use in small group activities and conversations.	
2) To understand and use vocabulary for joining sentences, e.g. when, because, until, unless, before, after.	2) Correct use in everyday speech on 8/10 separate occasions.	2) Reading books; picture books; posters; language cards; group discussions.	2) Talk about meanings of the words. Encourage correct use when discussing pictures etc.	2) Model correct use. Encourage correct use in small group activities and conversations.	
3) To spell 30 of the NLS Year 4/5 words.	3) Accurate when tested at random on three separate occasions.	3) Worksheets; cut up words; wooden/plastic letters; games; computer programs; initial letter clues for words in context.	3) Include the words in class spelling lists.	3) Play games to encourage spelling of the words.	
4) To show understanding of the text that has been read.	4) Answers comprehension questions accurately on three separate occasions.	4) Verbal questions; to formulate own questions based on text.	4) Ask relevant questions. Explain figures of speech.	4) Set comprehension work, e.g. worksheets to accompany reading books.	
5) To read and spell shortened forms of words using apostrophes.	5) Accurate on three separate occasions.	5) Games to match full words with contractions, e.g. dominoes; English textbooks.	5) Talk about the parts of the words replaced by the apostrophe.	5) Provide games and exercises to reinforce knowledge of shortened forms of words.	

Parents/carers need to: help to learn any words that are sent home. Talk about books with . . . .

Student needs to: Practise spelling the words. Remember to bring books back to school.

Guidelines for a Speech and Language Friendly School

51

Overall aims	Baselines	Targets for this term	√ / ✗	Actual outcome
To expand ███'s basic vocabulary.	███ uses a reduced range of adjectives.	To describe a range of items according to what they look like, feel like and sound like.		
To improve the clarity of ███'s speech.	███ substitutes the sounds 'k' 's' 'sh' and 'f' with a 'h' when the sounds are at the beginning of a word.	To produce the sounds 'k' 's' 'sh' and 'f' at the beginning of words in his natural, spontaneous speech.		
To improve ███'s ability to find the word he wants to say.	Can discriminate the sounds at the beginnings of words but struggles to think of the first sound of a word when he hasn't heard it.	To identify the first sound of a word (which he hasn't heard, e.g. he's seen the thing he's got to think about, but hasn't heard anybody name it).		
	Can confuse similar sounding words.	To describe items that have been grouped together because they have the same first sound, saying one main characteristic about each item, e.g. the group made is: table, tiger, tennis. ███ could say: • Table – you sit at it • Tiger – it's a wild animal • Tennis – it's a sport Try to guess the item from ███'s description. Guide him into giving good clues.		

Overall aims	Baselines	Targets for this term	√ / ✗	Actual outcome
To expand ███'s basic vocabulary.	███ uses a reduced range of adjectives.	To describe a range of items according to what they look like, feel like and sound like.		
To develop ███'s understanding of words in sentences.	███ doesn't understand the prepositions 'behind', 'in front', 'next to'.	To understand the prepositions 'behind', 'in front', 'next to' in sentences at a three key word level.		
	███ doesn't understand the past tense.	To consistently answer questions correctly about events that have already happened (in the recent past), e.g. Who has climbed the climbing frame? What did you have for lunch?		
To develop ███'s interaction skills.	███ initiates an interaction then doesn't respond to the response he receives, e.g. she will call your name, but when she's got your attention, she doesn't respond and continue the interaction.	To initiate an interaction and get a response, then continue the interaction by asking a question or commenting on something appropriate. To be observed on a number of occasions.		
To develop ███'s reasoning skills.	███ doesn't understand that a current situation exists because of something that has already happened.	To say what caused a situation to occur, e.g. Why are they wet? Why is the boy crying?		
To improve the clarity of ███'s speech.	███ substitutes the initial sounds 't' 'f' and 's' with 'h'.	To produce the sounds 't', 'f', and 's' at the beginning of words.		

Overall outcome for term: [**F** (fully achieved), **M** (mostly 70 – 100%), **P** (partially <70%), **N** (not 0%)]

Overall aims	Baselines	Targets for this term	√ / ✗	Actual outcome
To develop ■■'s production of sentences.	■■■ tends to omit the subject in a sentence when describing something.	To consistently use the pronouns 'I', 'you', 'he', 'she', 'they' when he's describing something.		
To improve the clarity of ■■'s speech.	■■■ only says one of the consonants in 's' blends at the beginning of words, e.g. 'poon' for 'spoon', 'tairs' for 'stairs'.	To produce both consonants in 's' blends at the beginning of words in his natural, spontaneous speech.		
To begin to develop his writing skills by sounding out cvc words.	■■■ to put his phonic knowledge to use by correctly spelling simple cvc words.	To begin by using aids to constructing cvc words, 'earobics' magnetic letters etc, then develop to writing them independently.		
To count forwards and backwards to 20 fluently. To know his number bonds to 10.	To know all numbers to 20 especially 11-20. Be able to count on and back from any number. Know which 2 numbers make 10 and do it practically.	To practise counting using practical as well as mental strategies to achieve fluency. To become increasingly faster at knowing his number bonds to 5 and then to 10.		

Overall aims	Baselines	Targets for this term	√ / ✗	Actual outcome
To expand ■■■'s basic vocabulary.	■■■ uses a reduced range of adjectives.	To describe a range of items according to what they look like, feel like and sound like.		
To develop ■■■'s understanding of words in sentences.	■■■ doesn't understand the prepositions 'behind', 'in front', 'next to'.	To understand the prepositions 'behind', 'in front', 'next to' in sentences at a three key word level.		
	■■■ doesn't understand the past tense.	To consistently answer questions correctly about events that have already happened (in the recent past), e.g. Who has climbed the climbing frame? What did you have for lunch?		
	■■■ doesn't understand negative sentences using 'not', or 'n't', e.g. Who isn't eating?	To understand negative sentences that use 'not' or 'n't', e.g. Who can't reach the pencil?		
To develop ■■■'s reasoning skills.	■■■ doesn't understand that a current situation exists because of something that has already happened.	To say what caused a situation to occur, e.g. Why are they wet? Why is the boy crying?		

Overall outcome for term: [**F** (fully achieved), **M** (mostly 70 – 100%), **P** (partially <70%), **N** (not 0%)]

Child-centred response form

Name	Date of birth
Arrival date at setting	Today's date

About the child

Medical needs/Previous concerns/Professionals involved?

Areas of ability (What can the child do?)

What are our concerns?

What has worked well when working with this child?

What shall we do next?

In our daily work with the child?	In communication with parents?

Do we need to contact anyone for support (i.e. outside agencies)?

If yes, who?

Date to review progress _____

References

There are a number of books and documents that have strongly influenced the authors' work. These include:

McMinn, J. (2002) *Supporting children with speech and language impairment and associated difficulties.* Birmingham: The Questions Publishing Company.

Speake, J. (2003) *How to identify and support children with speech and language difficulties.* Wisbech: LDA.

The Dyscovery Centre publications mentioned in the 'Books and resources' section.

Johnson, M. (2001) *Functional Language in the Classroom (and at home).* Manchester: Manchester Metropolitan University.

Stuart, L., Wright, F., Grigor, S. and Howey, A. (2002) *Spoken Language Difficulties: Practical Strategies and Activities for Teachers and Other Professionals.* London: David Fulton Publishers.

Books and resources

Expressive and receptive language

Books

Biddulph, L. and McQueen, D. *How to Help Talking.* First Community Health, Beecroft Clinic, Cannock Chase Hospital, Brunswick Road, Cannock, Staffordshire WS11 2XY.

Grauberg, E. (1998) *Elementary Mathematics and Language Difficulties: A book for teachers, therapists and parents.* London: Whurr Publications.

The Dyscovery Centre. A variety of publications, e.g. Super series of four booklets: *Activity, Listening and Attention, Helping the Child, Handwriting.*

Locke, A. *Living Language and Teaching Talking.* NFER Nelson.

Martin, D. and Miller, C. (1996) *Speech and Language Difficulties in the Classroom.* London: David Fulton.

McMinn, J. (2002) *Supporting Children with Speech and Language Impairment and Associated Difficulties.* Birmingham: The Questions Publishing Company.

Snowling, M. and Stackhouse, J. (1995) *Dyslexia, Speech and Language: A Practitioner's Book.* London: Whurr Publications.

Speake, J. (2003) *How to Identify and Support Children with Speech and Language Difficulties.* Wisbech: LDA.

Schroeder, A. (2001) *Time to Talk: A programme to develop oral and social interaction skills at Reception and KS1.* Wisbech: LDA.

Turnbull, J. and Stewart, T. (1996) *Helping Children Cope with Stammering.* Sheldon Press.

Resources

Earwiggo – a set of six books on rhythm, pitch and simple songs. Lovely Music, J 7 Westgate, North Yorkshire LS24 9JB.

Functional Language in the Classroom (and at home) by Maggie Johnson, available from The Commercial Office, Manchester Metropolitan University, Elizabeth Gaskell Site, Hathersage Road, Manchester M13 0JA (ideas and suggestions to improve listening and understanding).

Jolly Phonics materials – Jolly Learning Ltd., Tailours House, High Road, Chigwell, Essex.

LDA – a wide range of resources to help with many areas of speech and language work, e.g. *Language Cards, Listen and Do* etc. LDA, Duke Street, Wisbech, Cambs. PE13 2AE.

Ravensburger – games, e.g. *What's my name?* and *Tell a story.*

Sequencing stories – photocopiable sequencing materials from Learning Materials Ltd., Dixon Street, Wolverhampton WV2 2BX.

Speechmark Publishing – a range of books and products. www.speechmark.net

Winslow Press – a range of resources such as *Leap into Listening* (photocopiable listening activities). Winslow Press, Goytside Road, Chesterfield S40 2PH.

Glue Ear: Guidelines for Teachers – Hearing Research Trust.

Listening Skills: Early Years and Listening Skills KS1 – photocopiable sheets for listening activities. Birmingham: Questions Publishing.

What am I? – listening game (and other listening tapes). Early Learning Centre.

Social use of language skills

Books

Bliss, T. and Tetley, J. (1993) *Circle Time and Developing Circle Time.* Bristol: Lucky Duck Publishers.

Frances, J. and Brownsword, K. (1999) *A Positive Approach.* Belair.

Gray, C. (2000) *The New Social Story Book.* Arlington, USA: Future Horizons.

Martin, D. and Miller, C. (2003) *Speech and Language Difficulties in the Classroom.* London: David Fulton Publishers.

Mildred, M. (1989) *Let's Play Together.* Green Print.

Mortimer, H. (1998) *Learning Through Play – Circle Time.* Leamington Spa: Scholastic.

Moseley, J. (1996) *Quality Circle Time.* Wisbech: LDA.

Moseley, J. (1998) *More Circle Time.* Wisbech: LDA.

Sher, B. (1995) *Popular Games for Positive Play Therapy.* John Wiley & Sons.

Sher, B. (1998) *Self-Esteem Games.* John Wiley & Sons.

Resources

Mad, Sad, Glad game – 'emotions' photo-cards from Winslow Press (also available from LDA).

Superstickers – have badges such as 'I listen carefully'. PO Box 55, 4 Balloo Avenue, Bangor, County Down BT19 7PJ.

Social Skills posters – Good Listening; Good Talking; Good Waiting; Good Asking; Good Thinking. Taskmaster Ltd., Leicester.

The Giggly, Grumpy, Scary Book – a songbook with CD. Universal Edition, London.

Developmental co-ordination difficulties

Books

Dennison, P. and Dennison, G. (1992) *Brain Gym.* London: Body Balance Books.

Kirkby, A. (1999) *Dyspraxia: The Hidden Handicap.* Souvenir Press.

Macintyre, C. (2000) *Dyspraxia in the Early Years.* London: David Fulton Publishers.

Portwood, M. (1999) *Developmental Dyspraxia: Identification and Intervention. A manual for parents and professionals.* London: David Fulton Publishers.

Poustie, J. (1997) *Solutions for Specific Learning Difficulties.* Hitchin: Dyspraxia Foundation.

Russell, J.P. *Graded Activities for Children with Motor Difficulties.* Cambridge: Cambridge University Press.

Resources

Anything Left-Handed – a range of resources, 18 Avenue Road, Belmont, Surrey SM2 6JD.

Easylearn – good range of resources (enquiry@easylearn.co.uk).

Gymnic/Epsan Waterfly UK Ltd., Anglo House, Worcester Road, Stourport on Severn DY13 9AW.

LDA – has a large range of products and resources.

Rompa Ltd., Goytside Road, Chesterfield S40 2PH.

Happy Puzzle Company – puzzles and games (www.happypuzzle.co.uk).

Parents as part of the team

Books

Blamires, M., Robertson, C. and Blamires, J. (1997) *Parent Teacher Partnership.* London: David Fulton Publishers.

Gascoigne, E. (1995) *Working with Parents as Partners in SEN.* London: David Fulton Publishers.

Useful contacts

AFASIC – this is a parent-led organisation that works on behalf of children and young people who have a speech and language difficulty. AFASIC publishes a number of useful leaflets and booklets.
AFASIC, 2nd Floor, 50–52 Great Sutton Street, London EC1V ODJ
Telephone helpline: 0845 355 5577
Website: www.afasic.org.uk

ICAN – helps children with speech and language difficulties across the UK.
ICAN, 4 Dyer's Buildings, Holborn, London EC1N 2QP
Tel: 0845 225 4071
Website: www.ican.org.uk

Talking point – this is a website run by ICAN, AFASIC and RCSLT jointly for parents and teachers.
Website: www.talkingpoint.org.uk

The Dyscovery Centre – provides a specialist service with an interdisciplinary team helping individuals with learning difficulties.
The Dyscovery Centre, 4a Church Road, Whitchurch, Cardiff CF14 2DZ
Tel: 0292 062 8222
Website: www.dyscoverycentre.co.uk

The Dyspraxia Foundation – a national charity which has many leaflets, factsheets, books and software available.
The Dyspraxia Foundation, 8 West Alley, Hitchin, Hertfordshire SC5 1EG
Tel: 01462 454986
Website: www.dyspraxiafoundation.org.uk